ESSENTIAL OILS RECIPES ON A BUDGET

150+ From Health, Home, Pets & Aromatherapies to Medicines That Work!

by Oliver Kennedy

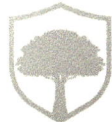

CLADD
PUBLISHING

Cladd Publishing Inc.
USA

This publication is designed to provide accurate information regarding the subject matter covered. It is sold with the understanding that neither the author nor the publisher is providing medical, legal or other professional advice or services. Always seek advice from a competent professional before using any of the information in this book. The author and the publisher specifically disclaim any liability that is incurred from the use or application of the contents of this book.

Essential Oils Recipes on a Budget: 150+ From Health, Home, Pets & Aromatherapies to Medicines That Work!

ISBN 978-1-946881-28-1 (e-book)
ISBN 978-1-946881-27-4 (paperback)

Contents

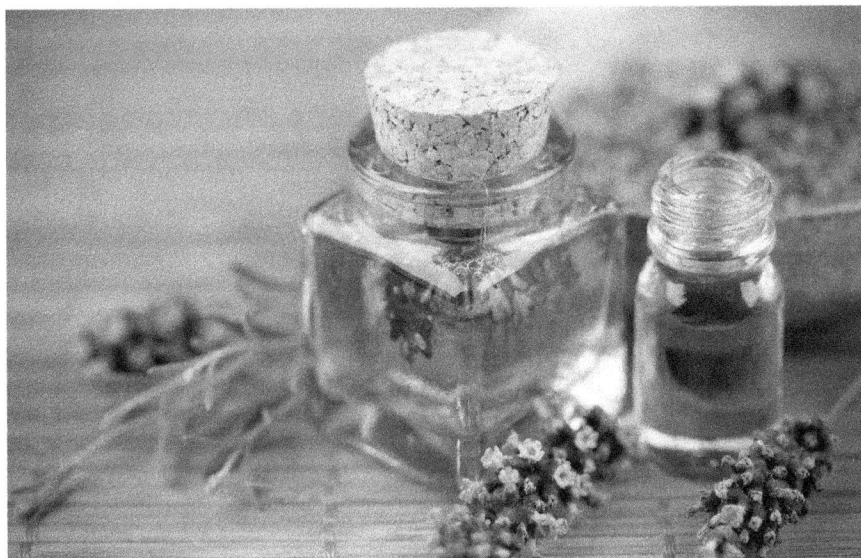

Essential Oils Q&A

Q: What does EO mean?

A: EO or EOs is the abbreviation for Essential Oils. It is commonly used and will be used throughout this book.

Q: Will I be able to use the EO recipes on a budget & with little experience?

A: Yes, the 150 EO recipes I have provided are budget friendly, non-toxic formulas for home, health and beauty. I also share the most versatile EOs for everyday use, and how they can be substituted or swapped out. This is an excellent book for normal people wanting to enhance their life with Essential Oils, but do not want to spend an erroneous amount of money and time learning techniques from scratch.

Q: Can I substitute EOs?

A: You can swap out oils or substitute for your favorite in almost all cases. Some of the most powerful essential oils for cleaning are lemon, lime, wild orange, thyme, peppermint, lavender, eucalyptus, melaleuca (Tea Tree), rosemary, and cinnamon. Mix and match as you wish.

Q: Glass Bottle or Plastic?

A: Essential oils can degrade plastic. That is way its recommended to store oils in glass. However, since you are not ingesting cleaning recipes, it would be fine to store those in a regular plastic spray bottle.

Q: Base product vs. Carrier Oil?

A: A base product is a cream, lotion, shampoo, gel or anything that has already been made. You can add a few drops of Essential Oils to enhance the product. A Carrier Oil is a pure oil, that is used to dilute the strength of EOs, and help prolong its aroma. As a rule of thumb, I wouldn't apply Essential Oils directly onto your skin without diluting it in a carrier oil first.

Although, there are some EOs that you can do this with, unless you are experienced avoid direct application. In addition to carrier oils, many times you will be diluting the oils in water as a spray, bath or soak.

Q: Can I ingest drops directly in my mouth?

A: Never ingest drops directly on your tongue or in your mouth without some sort of dilution. Essential Oils are powerful, it may take hundreds or thousands of plants and fruit to make one little jar. Be wise and follow a recipe that includes dilution prior to ingesting.

Q: Can I adjust the strength of the recipe?

A: Yes, you can and should limit the drops of EO based on your personal sensitivity towards the strength. Most recipes in this book are light-medium strength. However, you can always reduce or increase slightly in either direction unless stated.

Carrier Oils

The scent of EOs will evaporate quickly, unless combined with a carrier oil. Carrier oils usually come from the fatty portion of a plant and help the essential oils maintain their scent for long periods of time.

Carrier Oils are also important for diluting your EOs prior to ingesting or direct use on the skin.

These are Excellent Carrier Oils:
- Almond Oil
- Jojoba Oil
- Olive Oil
- Grapeseed Oil
- Avocado Oil
- Coconut Oil

Diluting Cheat Sheet

To dilute EOs, add them to, carrier oils, water, unscented bath oils, hand and body lotions, massage lotions and shower gels. Or use them directly on objects to provide beautiful room aromas. Do not use directly on skin unless stated.

- Massage: 3-5 drops per tsp. of base oil or lotion
- Inhalation: 1-2 drops in boiling water or on tissue paper
- Light Bulb Ring: 1-2 drops
- Bath: 5-10 drops in bath water
- Sauna: 1-2 drops to 2 ½ cups water
- Facial: 1-3 drops in base product
- Foot Bath: 5-8 drops in bowl of water
- Facial Sauna: 5-10 drops in bowl of water
- Cleanser: 10-20 drops in 4 ounces of base product
- Body: 5-12 drops in base product
- Chest Rub: 5-20 drops to 1 oz. of carrier oil
- Washing Machine: 5-20 drops per load
- Vacuum Cleaner: 5-10 drops
- Auto Vent Outlet: 1-3 drops
- Artificial Tree: 5-15 drops

10 EOs to Avoid

Some EOs are not safe for skin contact or ingestion. They can cause skin problems or may even be poisonous.

Avoid These Essential Oils:
- Bitter Almond
- Calamus
- Horseradish
- Mugwort
- Mustard
- Rue
- Yellow Camphor
- Savin
- Southernwood
- Tansy

10 EOs That Repel Bugs

Store bought bug-spray can be filled with harmful chemicals that should not be put on our bodies. The list below will help you repel most all bugs on your body or around your home. Use this list to mix and match or substitute Essential Oils found in my recipes.

Natural Oils That Provide Temporary Relief from Bugs:

- Castor oil
- Cedar oil
- Cinnamon oil
- Citronella oil
- Clove oil
- Geranium oil
- Lemon eucalyptus oil
- Lemongrass oil
- Peppermint oil
- Rosemary oil

10 EOs Easy to Cook With

1-3 drops of Essential Oils can go a long way. You should start off with 1 drop and increase as desired.

- Lemon (Add to anything that calls for lemon zest)
- Lime (marinades, salsa, tortilla soups, anything that calls for lime juice or lime zest)
- Wild Orange (Add to anything that calls for calls for orange zest
- Ginger (to replace fresh ginger)
- Cardamom (great addition to most drinks, sweets, baked goods, or coffee)
- Peppermint (great in brownies, or anything chocolate)
- Thyme (Add to anything that calls for thyme and you don't have the fresh herb)
- Cumin (great in soups, tacos, or chili)
- Dill (add to marinades, dressings or dips)
- Black Pepper (add to marinades or meats)

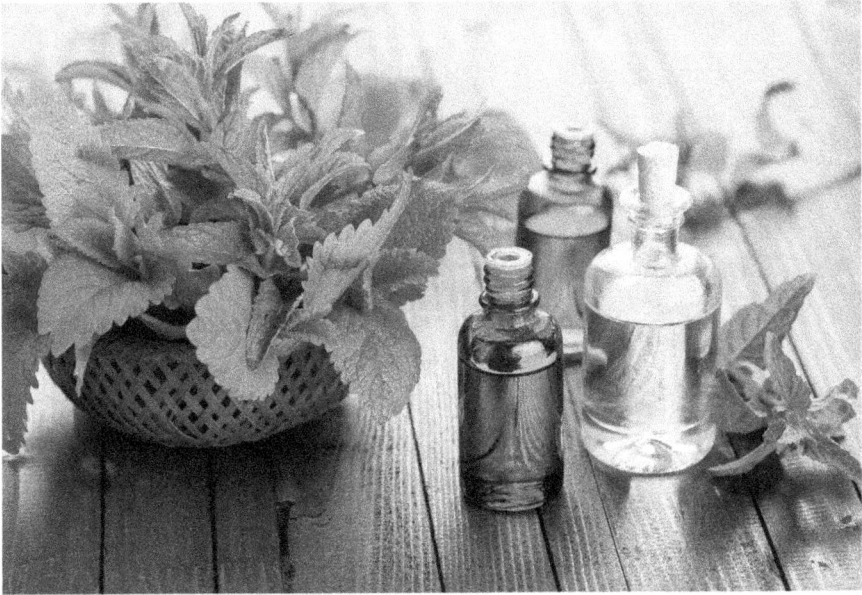

Must Have EO's

High quality Essential Oils can be expensive and overwhelming. The 10 essential oils listed below have a number of different benefits that range from health care to home and garden. But if you only want to have a few in the house at any given time, these are the most important.

Lavender

Lavender has been used for medicinal and home care purposes for thousands of years. It is by far the most versatile EOs you can get.

Commonly used for:
- Skin rashes
- Acne
- Insect bites

- Minor burns
- Soothing agent
- Relaxation
- Odor eliminator
- Disinfectant

A few drops of Lavender EO in a bath will soothe nerves and aid you in sleeping. It can be rubbed into your temples and forehead to relieve headaches with a carrier oil. In addition, a sachet of Lavender EO can keep moths away.

It's fantastic to use as odor control for laundry, stinky socks and sweaty gym clothes. Add Lavender EO to a mop bucket to super clean your floors

Tea Tree

Tea Tree is often called "the medicine cabinet in a bottle," as it can be used to treat almost any common ailment.

Commonly used for:
- Athlete's foot
- Dermatitis/eczema
- Acne
- Cold sores
- Nail fungus
- Warts
- Insect bites
- Disinfectant
- Bug repellant

You can add a few drops of it to unscented shampoo to alleviate dandruff, psoriasis, and head lice.

Lemon

This is the most versatile EO out there. It can be used for everything imaginable, and is very safe to use and ingest in the kitchen. I include Lemon EO in many of my everyday uses, foods, cleaners, therapeutics and medicine.

Commonly used for:
- Relieves bad breath
- Lessons dandruff
- Alleviates anxiety
- anti-microbial sanitizer
- Disinfectant cleaning agent
- Odor eliminator
- Lemon substitute for cooking

FYI: Lemon EO will make your skin photosensitive, so wait 12 hours before direct sun exposure.

Peppermint

Peppermint is much like lemon when it comes to the vast uses for this amazing EO.

- Alleviates nausea and an upset stomach
- Relieve stomach cramps and queasiness
- Draws out insect
- Relieve bronchial congestion
- Soothing
- Eliminate odors
- Antibacterial
- Deter rodents and spiders: they can't stand the scent of it

Eucalyptus

Eucalyptus comes from Australia, and is one of the few
Essential Oils that you should always have on hand.

Commonly used for:
- Alleviating chest congestion
- Eases asthma attacks
- Lessens the pain of fibromyalgia
- Reduces pain associated with the shingles speed the healing process
- Eliminate germs and odors
- Disinfectant

Clove

Clove EO has been used for dental issues for ever. It is
considered one of the best treatments available for toothaches,
gum disease, cold sores, and canker sores. It should always be
diluted, and used with caution on very- sensitive skin.

Commonly used for:
- Athlete's foot
- Prickly heat rash
- Wounds and cuts
- Fungal infections
- Insect bites or stings
- Bruises
- Ear aches (poured on a cotton swab and tucked just inside the ear canal)

- Repels Mosquitos, moths and fleas
- Odor remover

Chamomile

Chamomile EO has been used to sooth and calm since the Roman era.

Commonly used for:
- Boils
- Dry skin
- Eczema
- Dermatitis
- Acne
- Bee and wasp stings
- Cuts
- Bruises
- Soothing
- Relaxes
- Aids in sleep
- Stress, anxiety, depression reducer
- Eases PMS and menopause symptoms
- Repels mites and fleas

Frankincense

Frankincense has long been considered one of the most valuable Essential Oils of All time.

Commonly used for:

- Acne
- Warts
- Cuts and scrapes (it's a great disinfectant)
- Boils
- Scar tissue
- Cysts
- Insect bites
- Alleviates stress, anxiety, panic attacks
- Aids in sleeping, depression and insomnia
- Reduces headaches, migraines

Grapefruit

Grapefruit EO is uplifting and multi-purpose. However, like lemon, grapefruit can make your skin photosensitive, so refrain from direct sunshine for 12–24 hours after application.

Commonly used for:

- Swollen lymph nodes
- Oily skin and hair
- Cellulite
- Acne
- Migraines or tension headaches
- Deodorant
- Repels fleas
- Anti-bacterial
- Odor eliminator

Oregano

Oregano EO is anti-inflammatory, anti-fungal, anti-parasitic, anti-microbial, and antiseptic. It is great to use around the house and on your body. However, never use undiluted. The undiluted oil can cause skin irritation, so wear gloves if you're going to use it full strength for home cleaning purposes.

Commonly used for:
- Fungal infections
- Bruises
- Athlete's foot
- Sprains
- Arthritis pain
- Fibromyalgia
- Tendonitis
- Cysts
- Warts
- Candida
- Shingles
- Herpes
- Anti-bacterial
- Repels bugs, mites, lice and fleas

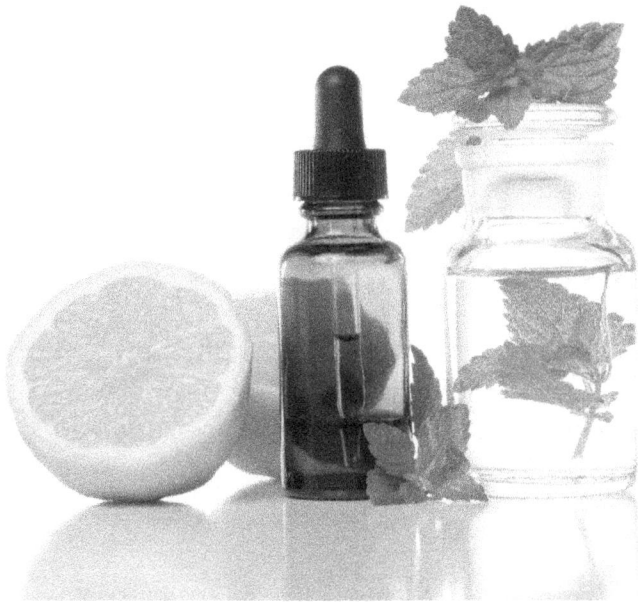

Aphrodisiac Oils

The following essential oils are excellent options to use as a perfume, or diluted in a carrier oil for a massaging oil. You can also add them to baths for a relaxing aroma.

Ylang Ylang

Ylang Ylang has a powerful floral aroma, and is an aphrodisiac. Add 3-5 drops per 1 ounce of carrier oil for a single massage. Has a feminine aroma.

Neroli

Neroli has a sweet floral aroma, which is very soothing to an overworked nervous system. Add 3-5 drops per 1 ounce of the chosen carrier oil. Has a feminine aroma.

Rose Absolute Bulgarian

This is a highly-prized EO and is one of the best aphrodisiacs. Rose has a deep floral aroma and is symbolic for the expression of love. Add 1-2 drops per 1 ounce of carrier oil. *Has a feminine aroma.*

Jasmine Absolute

Jasmine is an incredible aphrodisiac and sexual tonic. It is very calming to the mind and nervous system. It has deep, warm, floral notes. Add 1-2 drops per 1 ounce of carrier oil. *Has a feminine aroma.*

Sandalwood Australian

This has woody, balsamic, and earthy tones. Its aroma is valued for its ability to calm the mind. It is also used as a sexual tonic. To use in a massage oil, add 6-10 drops of Sandalwood per 1 ounce of the chosen carrier oil. *Has a masculine aroma.*

Patchouli

It is well-known for its aphrodisiac properties. Patchouli is very grounding and intoxicating to the senses. Add 1-2 drops per 1 ounce of carrier oil. Has a masculine aroma.

Vetiver

This warm, smoky, woody EO is very relaxing. It gently sedates an overworked mind. Add 2 drops per 1 ounce of carrier oil. Has a masculine aroma.

150+ Essential Oils Recipes On a Budget

On a Budget

In Alphabetical Order A-Z

Air Freshener

Sweet Lavender Air Freshener

Ingredients:

- 3/4 cup water
- 2 tablespoons vodka, rubbing alcohol, or real vanilla extract
- 10 drops lavender essential oil
- 5 drops chamomile essential oil

How To:

- Combine in an 8 oz. spray bottle
- Shake well
- Spray throughout the house to eliminate smells

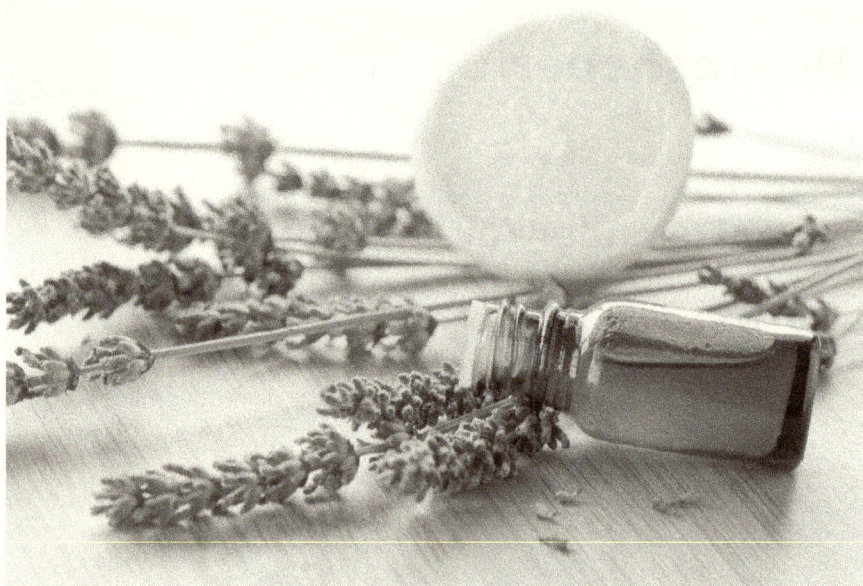

Alkalinity (pH) Of The Body

If you believe your body's acidity is high, here are quick remedies to use.

Signs of high body acidity (low pH) includes:
- Mucus buildup
- Joint pain
- Cold hands or feet
- Reduced sex drive
- Chemical sensitivity
- Heartburn
- Metallic taste in the mouth
- Muscular pain

Alkaline (pH) Booster

This remedy will help to balance pH levels in the body. It will also help with stomach acid and reduce acidosis.

Ingredients:
- ⅓ Teaspoons of baking soda
- 2 drops of Lemon EO
- 8 ounces of purified water

How To:
- Mix everything together
- Drink

Alkaline Water Enhancer

Drink Alkaline water all day long and feel alive.

How To:
- Add ½ a teaspoon of baking soda to a gallon of purified water
- Add 3-5 drops of Lemon EO
- Shake well
- Enjoy at your own leisure

Arts & Crafts

Play Dough

This is the best play dough recipe. Its identical to the store-bought brands, but it's completely non-toxic, gluten free, soy free, preservative free, food grade, and vegan.

Ingredients:
- 2 cups baking soda
- 1 cup cornstarch
- 1 ½ cups water
- 1 tablespoon oil
- 2-10 drops of any EO you like

FYI: Popular EO's for Play Dough are Lemon, Wild Orange and Peppermint or Wild Orange, and Lime.

How To:
- Combine all ingredients into a saucepan. Add your favorite EO after it starts to thicken
- Mix well
- Heat on the stove top over medium, stirring constantly
- The baking soda will fizz for a long time before it starts to thicken
- When thickening occurs, remove it from the heat immediately
- Add your favorite Essential Oils and mix
- Let cool, partially covered until you can handle it
- Separate into balls
- Add food coloring into the balls and knead

Smoke Smell Remover

Ashtray Odor Eliminator

This recipe eliminates the smell of heavily used ashtrays. The layer of soda traps the smoke from the ashes and discarded butts.

How To:
- Fill the bottom of an ashtray with baking soda
- Add 3-5 drops of your favorite EO
- Use as usual

FYI: The most popular EOs for this purpose are Bergamot, Grapefruit, Lemon, Lemongrass, Lime, Mandarin, Orange, Sage, and Tangerine.

Smoke Odor Spray

If you smoke or live next to someone who does, you can easily eliminate the smell of cigarette smoke with a few drops of essential oils.

How To:
- Add four drops of Rosemary
- 4 drops Tea Tree
- 4 Eucalyptus essential oils in a spray bottle
- Fill up with water
- Shake well
- Spray anywhere you can smell smoke odor

Athletes Foot

Fungal Foot Soak

Ingredients:
- 5 drops of Tea Tree oil
- 1 drop of Lemon oil
- 1 tablespoon of baking soda
- 1 tablespoon of Epsom salt
- 2 tablespoons of cider vinegar

How To:
- Mix all the ingredients in a bowl of warm water
- Soak your feet for 5-15 minutes
- Dry your feet with a clean cloth

Fungal Dab

Ingredients:
- 2 drops of Cypress essential oil
- 25 drops of Lavender essential oil
- 30 drops of Tea tree oil

How To:
- Blend all the ingredients and keep the mix in a dark-colored glass bottle
- Add 2 drops on a cotton swab
- Dab between the toes and around the toenails

Baby

Relieve Diaper Rash

This is an excellent way to relieve your baby's diaper rash naturally.

Ingredients:
- 1/4 cup virgin coconut oil
- 15 drops Lavender EO
- 10 drops Tea Tree EO
- Saucepan
- Glass storage container

How To:
- Slightly melt coconut oil
- Add Lavender and Melaleuca essential oils
- Store in glass container
- Wash and dry the affected area
- Gently rub mixture into skin
- A small amount goes a long way

Clean Cloth Diapers

How To:
- Dissolve 1/2 cup of baking soda
- 5 drops of Lavender EO in 2 quarts of water
- Soak diapers thoroughly for up to 8 hours
- Wash as usual

Bathroom

All-Purpose Cleaner with Lemon

Ingredients:
- 2 cups white vinegar
- 2 cups water
- 1 teaspoon natural dish soap (NOT castile soap)
- 30 drops Lemon EO
- 20 drops Tea Tree EO

How To:
- Mix all ingredients in a quart-sized spray bottle
- Shake to combine
- Spray and wipe anywhere

Mint Glass Cleaner

Ingredients:
- 3 cups distilled water
- 1/4 cup rubbing alcohol or vodka
- 1/4 cup vinegar
- 20 drops Peppermint or Spearmint EO

How To:
- Combine all ingredients in a quart-sized spray bottle
- Shake to combine

- Spray on mirrors, windows, or stainless steel
- Wipe off with paper towels or old newspaper

Simple Citrus Soft Scrub

Ingredients:
- 1 cup baking soda
- 1/4 cup liquid castile soap
- 10 drops Lemon EO
- 10 drops Lime EO
- 10 drops Wild Orange EO

How To:
- Mix ingredients together to form a paste (add more castile soap if needed)
- Apply with rag or sponge
- Then rinse with clean water

Deep Clean Toilet Scrub

Ingredients:
- 1/2 cup baking soda
- 1/3 cup liquid dishwashing soap
- 1/4 cup hydrogen peroxide
- 30 drops Eucalyptus EO
- 3/4 cup water

How To:
- Mix together in a squeeze-type bottle, then squirt into toilet

- Scrub and let stand 20 minutes
- Flush the toilet to rinse

Daily Shower Spray

Ingredients:
- 1.5 cups water
- 1 cup white vinegar
- 1/2 cup rubbing alcohol
- 1 teaspoon natural liquid dish soap (not castile soap)
- 15 drops Lime EO
- 15 drops Tea Tree EO

How To:
- Combine in a quart-sized spray bottle
- Spray daily on shower door and walls after use

Bathroom Scrub

Make a bathroom scrub that works wonders.

How To:
- Mix 1 cup baking soda with 1 tablespoon dishwashing soap
- Add vinegar until it reaches a creamy texture
- Add 2-5 drops of any citrus EO
- Use throughout your entire bathroom and kitchen

Tub Cleaning Gel

Ingredients:
- 1 cup white vinegar
- 1/2 cup dishwashing liquid
- Squeeze bottle
- 15 drops Tea Tree EO
- 10 drops Sweet Orange EO

How To:
- Heat the vinegar in a small saucepan on the stove until hot (but not boiling)
- Carefully stir the dishwashing soap in until combined
- Take off heat and allow to cool slightly
- Add Essential Oils and mix
- Pour into the squeeze bottle
- Squirt onto shower and tub, and allow to sit for 1-3 hours
- Wipe off with a scrubber or sponge
- Rinse well

Toilet Fizzy Drops

Freshen things fast with toilet fizzy drops. They clean and eliminate smells immediately. Stash in a cute glass jar or container on the back of your toilet and simply drop in a fizzy when needed. It removes bad smells, clean your bowl, and is good for the septic. It's a miracle!

The next time things get smelly, after flushing, drop in a fizzy.

Ingredients:

- 1 cup baking soda
- 1/4 cup citric acid
- 1/2 teaspoon vinegar
- 1 tablespoon hydrogen peroxide
- 15 to 20 drops of any Essential Oils
- Sheet pan
- Parchment paper
- Measuring spoons
- Spray bottle (optional)

How To:

- Add baking soda to a mixing bowl – break up any clumps
- Add the citric acid
- In a small glass bowl, mix together the vinegar and hydrogen peroxide
- Now drop by drop, add the vinegar and hydrogen peroxide to the baking soda/citric acid mix
- If you add the liquid all at once, you'll have a huge mess
- Now add the essential oil and gently mix
- Great options are Wintergreen, Lemongrass, or Lavender
- Use a ½ teaspoon to scoop and mold the mixture into small half rounds
- tap the scoop onto a parchment-covered sheet pan
- You can spritz the rounds with equal parts vinegar and water to create a crust, it helps hold them together
- Let dry overnight
- Place the dried fizzy drops in a sealable glass jar or sturdy container
- Use as often as you would like
- Makes around 30 small fizzy drops

FYI: Its very decorative to place a label on the jar! And so that people don't think they are breath mints.

Septic Care

Regular use of baking soda and Essential Oils in your drains can help keep your septic system flowing. It will help maintain a favorable pH in your septic tank.

How To:
- Add toilet fizzy drops on a regular basis

Clean Shower Curtains

Clean and deodorize your vinyl shower curtain.

How To:
- Mix baking soda and Wild Orange (or any citrus)
- Add water to make a paste
- Scrub the shower curtain
- Rinse clean
- Hang it up to dry

Unclog a Shower Head

How To:
- Mix 1/3 cup of baking soda with 1 cup of white vinegar and 5 drops of Pine EO
- Pour into a thick freezer plastic bag

- Secure the bag over your dirty showerhead with a strong rubber band
- Leave the bag on the showerhead for 24-48 hours
- Remove the bag and wipe down with a warm cloth

FYI: You can also remove the shower head and place it into the plastic bag on the counter.

Bedroom

Fresh Linen Spray

Ingredients:
- 1/4 cup distilled water
- 3 tablespoons Witch Hazel or vodka
- 20 drops Lavender EO
- 15 drops Frankincense EO

How To:
- Add all ingredients to a small spritzer
- Shake well
- Spray on sheets, pillowcases, and linens

Freshen Closets

For fresh clothes, shoes and accessories use this trick.

How To:
- Place a box of baking soda on the shelf open
- Add 5 drops of your favorite EO to the top of the lid

Freshen Stuffed Animals

Keep favorite stuffed toys fresh with a dry shower of baking soda and EO.

How To:
- Add 2 drops of your favorite EO to ½ cup of baking soda
- Sprinkle baking soda on each stuffed toy
- Let sit for 1 hours
- Vacuum, shake or brush it off

Freshen a Musty Mattress

Refresh your mattress with this trick.

How To:
- Add 10 drops of your favorite EO for every ½ cup of baking soda
- Sprinkle all over your mattress
- Leave on for up to 4-24 hours
- Vacuum well

Bug Bites

If it Burns, Stings or Itches

For instant relief from bug bites use this elixir.

How To:
- Mix 2 tsp. baking soda
- 2 drops Lavender EO
- Place mixture on bite until dry
- Wash off with a warm damp towel
- Reapply as needed

Carpet & Rugs

Lemon Carpet Refresher

Ingredients:
- 1 cup baking soda
- 30 drops lemon essential oil

How To:
- Combine in a small container, and cover tightly with a lid
- Shake well
- Sprinkle on stale or smelly carpet and allow it to sit overnight
- Vacuum up the next morning

Outdoor Rugs

Ingredients:
- 1 box of baking soda
- 25 drops Lemon or Peppermint EO

How To:
- Combine in a small container, and cover tightly with a lid
- Shake well
- Sprinkle on outdoor rug or carpet
- Let sit overnight
- Vacuum or shake off

Super Absorber: Oil, Grease, Juice, & Wine Stains

Works On:
- Carpet
- Rugs
- Upholstery
- Linens
- Drapes
- Blankets
- Concrete
- Hard floors
- Chair cushions and more...

How To:
- Mix 1 cup of baking soda
- 20 drops of Cinnamon Leaf EO
- Sprinkle a heavy amount directly on the liquid stain
- Let the soda sit until the liquid has absorbed
- Use a paper towel or dry cloth to remove the baking soda off the stained surface
- Now you can use a warm wet cloth by itself, or a spot cleaner to remove left over residue
- When completely dry, vacuum, wash or sweep the area well

Colds – Flu – Allergies

Congestion & Cough Relief Balm

At night when ready for bed.

Ingredients:
- 1 Tbsp. unrefined coconut oil
- 8 drops Eucalyptus EO
- 5 drops Lavender EO
- 2 drops Thyme EO

How To:
- Mix ingredients well
- Rub approximately a teaspoon-size amount over your chest area and go to bed
- Store in dark jar in cool place

Original Thieves Oil

Thieves Oil is an old Essential Oil recipe that was used during the Black Death of 1348. The EO combination blocks the protein synthesis of the virus, stopping it from spreading. This is an excellent choice for the flu season.

How To:
- Add 6 tsp. Olive Oil
- 15 drops Clove EO
- 10 drops Lemon EO

- 8 drops Cinnamon Bark EO
- 7 drops Eucalyptus EO
- 6 drop Rosemary EO
- Mix together
- Rub gently on your skin for relief or prevention

Cooking

Tea Perfection

How To:
- Use 1-2 drops Lemon or Orange EO for a perfect tea

Produce Wash

Most of our fresh produce is sprayed with some sort of chemical cocktail. It is very important to your health that you wash your fruits and vegies before consuming them.

How To:
- Add 2 drops of Lemon EO into a bowl of cool water
- Stir produce around with your hands
- Use a wash cloth to scrub root vegetables
- Let sit for 2 minutes
- Rinse in cool water
- Pat dry with a clean cloth or paper towel

Deodorant

Most ingredients used in store-bought deodorants are toxic.

Toxic Ingredients in Store-Bought Deodorant:
- Aluminum –This is a metal which has been linked to breast cancer in women, and an increased risk of Alzheimer's.
- Parabens –Paraben exposure has also been linked to birth defects and organ toxicity.
- Propylene glycol – This is a petroleum based material and damages the central nervous system, liver, and heart.
- Phthalates – Phthalates have been linked to a variety of health issues including birth defects.
- Triclosan – This chemical is disturbingly classified as a pesticide by the FDA.

For All Skin Types – Even Sensitive

Making your own deodorant is not only simple, but also safe for the entire family.

Ingredients:
- 1/3 cup coconut oil
- 2 Tbsp. of baking soda (reduce slightly for really sensitive skin)
- 1/3 cup arrow root powder
- 12 drops total of any EO (You can make a plain batch, then add oils based on individual preferences)
- Small flat mason jars

How To:

- Mix the coconut oil, baking soda, and arrow root powder together in a bowl
- Cream together the ingredients until it is similar to deodorant
- Mix in essential oils
- Put mixture into a small flat glass jar
- To use simply swipe two fingers gently into the mixture and rub on your underarms
- Wait two minutes before dressing to avoid any smearing on your clothes

FYI: Patchouli, Sandalwood, Oakmoss, Bay, Cypress, Ginger, Black Pepper, Vanilla, Vetiver, and the citrus oils are strongly favored by men. Popular feminine essential oils are Rose, Jasmine, Geranium, Clary Sage, Sweet Orange, Lemon or Grapefruit. However, you can add any oil or combination that makes you feel happy.

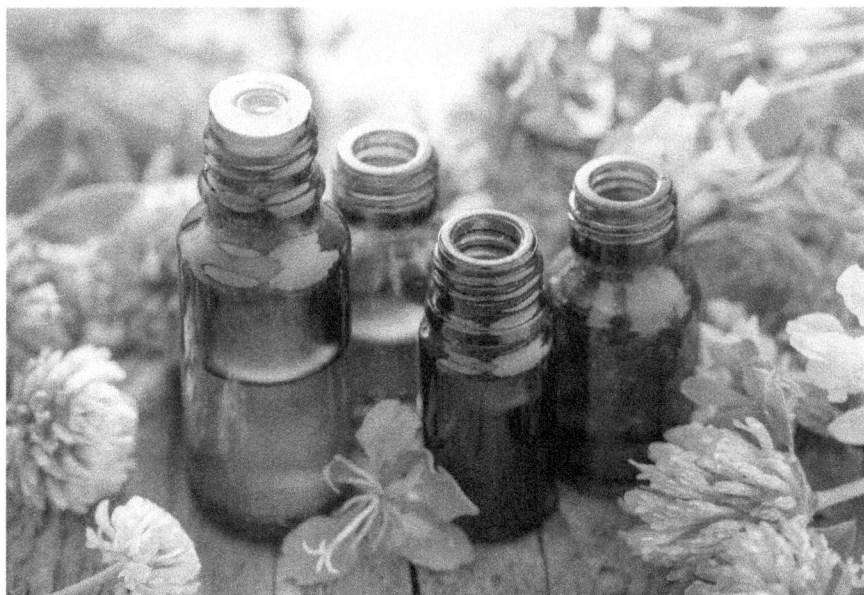

Facemask

Having a quality facemask to rescue your skin is essential. This will brighten your overall complexion, fade dark spots, gently exfoliates, softens skin, and is a natural antibacterial agent.

Brightening Facemask

Ingredients:
- 1/2 lemon fresh squeezed lemons (or 1 teaspoon of lemon juice from a bottle)
- 1 drop Lavender EO
- 1 or 2 tablespoons of baking soda
- 1 teaspoon of honey

How To:
- Mix all ingredients together in a small dish

- You should end up with a paste-like consistency
- Add more baking soda to thicken
- Wash off all makeup, dirt, and debris with your regular face wash
- Pat skin dry
- Apply the mask to your face and neck using circular motions
- Leave on your skin for 5-15 minutes
- You should feel some tingling and tightening of the mask
- If your skin starts to burn, remove the mask immediately
- Remove the mask with a lukewarm washcloth
- Close your pores! Use the coldest water you can handle, and pat it across your face
- Moisturize
- Use 1x per week or less

Furnace

Turn the Furnace into a Diffuser

How To:
- Put a few drops of Essential Oil on your furnace filter
- When the furnace blows air over the filter the essential oils will be diffused throughout your home
- Reapply every couple of days

Furniture

Gently Clean

How To:
- 1 Tbsp. baking soda
- 1-2 drops Lemon EO
- Add enough water to make a paste
- Rub lightly on surface
- Dry with a clean cloth

It Also Erases:
- Crayon
- Pencil
- Ink
- Furniture scuffs from painted surfaces

Marble Solution

Properly cleaning marble countertops, furniture or floors can be challenging. This is a wonderful recipe that will bring back its luster.

How To:
- Add 3 tablespoons of baking soda
- 2 drop Lemon EO
- 2 drops Lavender EO
- 1 quart of warm water
- Gently wash using a towel or soft sponge

- Dry with a clean cloth

Water Rings

Get rid of water rings on your tables with this mix.

How To:
- Mix 2 tsp. baking soda
- 1 drop Pine EO
- And enough toothpaste to make a paste
- Gently message the mix into the table in circular motions
- When done wipe with a damp cloth

Goo Remover

Lemon Goo Gone

Ingredients:
- 2 drops Lemon EO
- 2 tablespoons fractionated coconut oil or almond oil

How To:
- Mix together, then apply directly to sticker residue, random goo, gum, crayon marks, etc.
- Rub in with your fingers, then wipe away with a clean rag
- Repeat as needed

Hair Care

Chlorine Damaged Hair

After you have finished swimming, this spray will neutralize the damaging effects of the chlorine.

How To:
- Add 1 tbsp. of baking soda
- 2 drops Lavender EO
- 2 Drops Wild Orange EO
- to a small spray bottle and fill it with water
- Shake well
- Spritz on wet hair
- Shampoo and condition as usual

Remove Dandruff

How To:
- Mix 2 drops Chamomile EO with 1/8 cup baking soda
- massaging your wet scalp with a handful before shampooing
- Condition and rinse as usual

Clean Brushes & Combs

Remove oil build-up and hair product grime.

How To:

- Add 1 teaspoon of baking soda
- 5 drops Lemon EO
- 2 cups of warm water
- Drop brushes in mixture for up to 6 hours
- Rinse and allow to dry

Dry Shampoo Alternative

Use this dry shampoo alternative for crazy morning, greasy gym aftermath, and for hot summer days.

How To:

- Mix 2 drops Eucalyptus EO with 1/8 cup baking soda
- Sprinkle onto your roots
- Tousle your hair
- Then brush it to perfection

For Dry or Damaged Hair

How To:

- Add 10 drops Lavender EO
- 15 drops Rosemary EO
- 10 drops Tea Tree EO
- 2 tablespoons Sweet Almond oil
- 1 cup distilled water
- 1 cup liquid castile soap (unscented)
- 1 tablespoon Vitamin E oil
- Mix well and use

Oily Hair

How To:

- Add 15 drops of Basil EO
- 25 drops of Tea Tree EO
- 2 tablespoons Grapeseed EO
- 1/4 cup distilled water
- 1/4 cup liquid castile soap (unscented)
- 1 cup honey
- 1 tablespoon Vitamin E oil
- Mix well

Fine Hair

How To:

- Add 20 drops Chamomile Roman EO
- 20 drops Lavender EO
- 15 drops Tea Tree EO
- 2 tablespoons Sweet Almond oil
- 1 can coconut milk (unflavored, unsweetened)
- 1 cup liquid castile soap (unscented)
- 1 tablespoon Vitamin E oil
- Mix well

Hand Sanitizer

Peppermint Dream

Ingredients:
- 12 drops Lavender EO
- 6 drops Peppermint EO
- 3 ounces Aloe Vera gel
- 1 ounce grain alcohol
- 1 capsule of Vitamin E (400 IUs)

How To:
- First, mix together the oils and alcohol
- Then, add the Aloe Vera gel
- Pour the mixture into a bottle
- Shake before each use

Hard Floors

Bring Back Luster

To brighten a dull floor, try this gentle but effective solution.

How To:
- Dissolve ½ cup baking soda
- 10-20 Pine EO
- In a bucket of warm water
- Mop and rinse for a shiny floor

Headache Relief

Tension Headaches & Migraines

Use this inhalation method for a strong dose of EOs.

How To:
- Add 2 Lavender EO
- 2 Rose EO
- 2 Melissa EO
- You can inhale the oils from a tissue, a portable inhaler or add them to a diffuser

Temple Rub

How To:
- Add 1 drop of either Lavender, Rose or Melissa EO with 1 teaspoon of coconut oil
- Any carrier oil you have on hand will work fine
- Gently rub on temples and forehead

Shoulder & Neck Oil

How To:
- Add 4 drops Lavender EO
- 4 drops Peppermint EO
- 4 drops Marjoram EO

- Combined in 5 tsp of your preferred carrier oil (coconut, sesame, sweet almond, jojoba, grapeseed, macadamia)

Tension Headache Bath

This is a great way to release tension from your back, shoulders and neck area. The EO combination is excellent after a long day at work, or right before bed.

How To:
- 2 drops Lavender EO
- 3 drops Chamomile EO
- 3 drops Rose EO
- Run a warm bath, add all ingredients and soak.

Hives & Other Rashes

Soothing Hive Cream

How To:
- Combine 5 drops of German Chamomile EO in 1 ounce of coconut oil
- Apply to the hives after cleaning the affected area
- Store in a clean glass jar

Skin Inflammation Balm

How To:
- Place an ounce of raw Shea Butter in a small mason jar.
- Place the mason jar in a pan filled with a couple inches water.
- Slowly heat until the Shea Butter softens
- Remove from heat
- Mix in 5 drops of Myrrh EO
- Leave it to harden for an hour before use
- Apply to affected areas

Holiday Room Spray

These Essential Oils sprays smell absolutely wonderful, and aid your immune system in fighting seasonal colds.

Trim the Tree

How To:
- 16 oz. spray bottle
- 8 oz. distilled water
- 2 oz. Witch Hazel
- 12 drops Cinnamon EO
- 11 drops Orange EO
- 18 drops White Fir EO

Frosty Morning

How To:
- 16 oz. spray bottle
- 8 oz. distilled water
- 2 oz. Witch Hazel
- 23 drops Peppermint EO
- 23 drops Orange EO

Chai Wonderland

How To:
- 16 oz. spray bottle
- 8 oz. distilled water

- 2 oz. Witch Hazel
- 20 drops Orange EO
- 5 drops Nutmeg EO
- 5 drops Cinnamon EO
- 4 drops Clove EO
- 5 drops Cardamom EO

Perfect Peppermint

How To:
- 16 oz. spray bottle
- 8 oz. distilled water
- 2 oz. Witch Hazel
- 27 drops Peppermint EO
- 18 drops Ylang Ylang EO

Spice & Everything Nice

How To:
- 16 oz. spray bottle
- 8 oz. distilled water
- 2 oz. Witch Hazel
- 18 drops Bergamot EO
- 8 drops Ginger EO
- 8 drops Cassia EO
- 7 drops White Fir EO

By the Fire

How To:
- 16 oz. spray bottle
- 8 oz. distilled water
- 2 oz. Witch Hazel
- 12 drops Douglas Fir EO
- 13 drops Cassia EO
- 14 drops Orange EO
- 4 drops Clove EO

Zesty Gathering

How To:
- 16 oz. spray bottle
- 8 oz. distilled water
- 2 oz. Witch Hazel
- 17 drops Orange EO
- 8 drops Clove EO
- 8 drops Rosemary EO

Apple Pie

How To:
- 16 oz. spray bottle
- 8 oz. distilled water
- 2 oz. Witch Hazel
- 18 drops Orange EO
- 10 drops Cinnamon EO
- 10 drops Ginger EO

Gingerbread Man

How To:

- 16 oz. spray bottle
- 8 oz. distilled water
- 2 oz. Witch Hazel
- 18 drops Ginger EO
- 8 drops Cinnamon EO
- 8 drops Clove EO
- 4 drops Nutmeg EO

Jewelry

Natural Jewelry Cleaner

How To:

- 1 cup of very warm water
- 2 Tbsp. of baking soda
- 1 tsp. Witch Hazel
- 3 drops Lemon EO
- Then drop in your jewelry
- You can also use a soft bristle brush to remove grime
- Rinse in cool water and pat dry

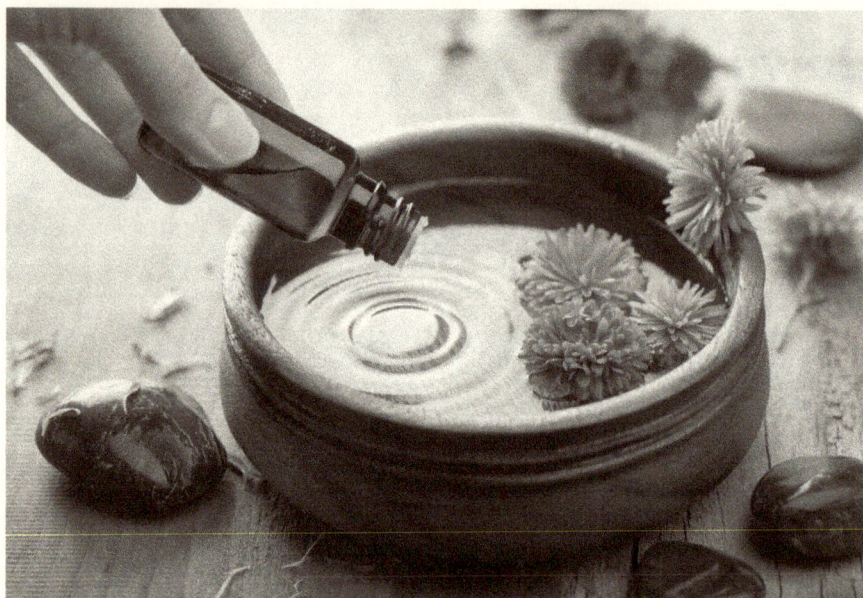

Kitchen

Clean the Machines

Dishwasher Clean

Clean the dishwasher and coffeemaker with these tricks.

How To:
- Add 1 tablespoon of baking soda
- 10 drops Lemon EO
- Run the dishwasher through a full cycle with NO dishes
- When completed, use like normal

Coffee-Pot Machine Clean

How To:
- Fill your coffee pot with warm water
- Add 1 tablespoon of baking soda and 3 drop Orange EO to the water
- Run the coffee-pot machine through a full cycle with NO coffee grounds
- When completed, run another full cycle with water only
- Then use like normal

Window, Glass, Shining Surface

How To:
- Add equal parts water to equal parts vinegar (white distilled)
- 4 drops of Lavender or Lemon EO per 4 oz. of liquid
- 1 drop of natural unscented dish soap per 4 oz. of liquid
- Pour into a spray bottle
- Use to safely clean the entire home

Stainless Steel Appliances

Magically clean any stainless-steel appliance, BBQ grill, refrigerator, microwave, sink, dishwashers, faucets, handles and more. You will never waste your money buying the store-bought cleaner ever again. Its non-toxic, and completely safe for the entire family.

How To:

- In a small mason jar add 1/4 cup Olive Oil and 2 drops Lemon EO
- Shake well
- Dip a dry cloth into mixture
- Wipe down any stainless steel in or around the home

FYI: if you do not want the aroma of an EO, then use Olive Oil by itself.

Shine Brass

Restore brass to its original beauty naturally with a thick paste.

How To:

- Mix 1 cup vinegar
- 2 tablespoons salt
- 4 drops of any citrus EO
- small amount of all-purpose flour
- Smear paste into the brass and rub it in with a dry sponge
- After it dries, rinse in warm water
- Polish to a shine

Deodorize the Cutting Board

If your cutting board is looking and smelling a little funky, this one is for you.

How To:

- Mix ½ cup baking soda
- 2 drops Lemongrass EO

- Sprinkle the cutting board, scrub, rinse
- Dry with a clean towel, let sit in an open-air location until completely dry

Baked on Grime

Everyone at one moment in time, makes a wonderful dish that destroys their nice pans. Don't soak for days and still never get it completely clean, use this wonderful and quick method.

How To:
- Fill your dish up with hot water
- Add a generous sprinkle of baking soda
- Add a good squirt of dishwashing soap
- Add 5 drops of Lemon EO
- Let sit for 15 minutes and wash as usual

Drain Deodorizer

Read caution before attempting this drain deodorizer. It is a very powerful cleaner!

Caution
- Use this method only if your pipes are metal
- Never mix with other cleaning solutions
- Don't use this if you have recently used a commercial drain product

How To:
- Add 10 drop Pine EO to ½ cup baking soda

- Pour mixture down the drain
- Add ½ cup vinegar down the drain
- After 15 minutes, slowly pour hot water down the drain (it likes to fizz)

Oven Cleaner Degreaser

Easy and non-toxic way to clean your oven.

How To:
- Sprinkle baking soda in your oven
- Make a spray with 1 cup water and 20 drops Lemon
- Spray the inside of the oven
- Let it sit overnight
- Mix a small bowl of warm water and a little dishwashing soap
- Then scrub the oven and remove clumps
- Finish with a clean damp wash cloth

Remove Refrigerator Odor

This is the most common usage and the easiest way to keep your refrigerator smelling odorless.

How To:
- Place an open box of baking soda in the door
- Place 2 drops of Grapefruit or Lemongrass EO on the lid
- Leave in the refrigerator door
- Add a few drops ever 2 weeks

Trash Can Odor Control

Everyone has a trashcan that could use some odor control. This is a great way to tame the smell.

How To:
- Add 5 drops Tea Tree EO
- 5 drops Lemon EO
- ½ cup of baking soda
- Sprinkle baking soda mixture on the bottom of your trashcan

Freshen Sponges

Sponges are often a forgotten source of germs. Clean often and well.

How To:
- Mix 4 tablespoons of baking soda in 1 quart of warm water
- Add 2 drops Lavender EO
- Add 2 drops Orange EO
- Soak stale-smelling sponges for 4-6 hours
- Rinse well with warm water, and let sit in an open-air location until completely dry

Clean the Microwave

This recipe works on even the messiest microwave.

How To:
- Add 2 Tbsp. of baking soda to ½ cup of warm water

- Add 10-15 drops of Pine EO
- Mix well
- Scrub inside and outside of the microwave
- Rinse with warm water

Deodorize Recyclables

Use this trick to remove smells from reusable containers.

How To:
- Mix baking soda and dishwashing soap together
- Add 1-3 drops Cypress or Lemongrass EO
- Clean using warm water – do not use HOT water if working with plastics
- Rinse well and dry

Deodorize Garbage Disposals

It's important to deodorize your garbage disposals 1x per month or more.

How To:
- Mix 20 drops Eucalyptus EO in 1/4 cup of baking soda
- Pour the mixture down the drain, while running warm tap water
- Turn on the disposal until all baking soda is washed away

Glassware Shine

This is a quick fix to shine dull, spotty glassware.

How To:
- Add a pinch of baking soda
- 5 drops of Lemon EO
- 1 cups of water in a spray bottle
- Shake and spray
- Can leave on up to 30 minutes
- Wipe your glassware with a dry cloth

Laundry & Clothes

Dry Cleaning

How To:
- Put 2 to 4 drops of EO on a clean cotton washcloth
- toss that washcloth into the dryer on along with the clothing to be freshened
- Run through dryer on fluff cycle
- Your clothes will smell and feel fresh

New Clothes Detox

Remove the harmful chemical finishes on new clothing.

How To:
- Add 1/2 cup of baking soda
- 5 drops of Lavender EO
- Mix with your regular detergent
- Wash clothes like normal

T-Shirt Grease Stain Remover

remove grease stains with Lemon Essential Oil.

How To:
- Put a few drops of Lemon EO on the grease stain
- Gently rub the fabric together

- Toss it into the wash
- Repeat as many times as needed
- Good on most fabrics

Brighten

This is a great way to get clothes cleaner and brighter.

How To:
- Add 1 cup of baking soda
- 5 drops of Lemon EO in the wash with your laundry detergent
- Wash clothes like normal – for whites, use warm/hot water

Rid Sneaker Smell

This trick will absorb the odor without making a mess, or harming delicate materials like suede.

How To:
- Add 2 drops of Tea Tree EO
- 2 drops Lavender EO on to a paper coffee filter, tissue paper, or cotton ball
- Stick it into a stinky shoe

Clean and Freshen Sports Gear

Clean Smelly Equipment:
- Mix 4 tablespoons baking soda in 1 quart warm water
- Add 5-15 drops Lemon or Lavender

- Gently scrub or soak to deodorize smelly sports equipment

Safely Clean Golf Irons:
- Mix 3 parts baking soda to 1 part water
- 2 drops Lemon or Eucalyptus EO
- Use a cloth or soft bristle brush to clean
- Rinse thoroughly
- Pat dry with a clean cloth

Clothes Iron Cleaner

Remove all the residue from your iron, so you do not get stains on light colored clothing.

How To:
- Mix a paste made from a little baking soda and vinegar
- Add 1 drop Pine or Lemon EO
- Gently rub onto the iron, making sure to avoid the holes
- Wipe the mixture off with a warm damp cloth

Lawn & Garden

Protect Garden from Hungry Animals

Easy and safe way to prevent animals and bugs from eating your garden.

How To:
- Mix 20 drops Peppermint EO
- Per 1 small box baking soda
- Shake well
- Scatter baking soda mix around garden beds

Lips

Plumper Pout

Your lips will feel slightly tingly and look fuller.

How To:
- Add 1-2 drops of peppermint essential oil to a tube of lip gloss
- Mix well using the lip gloss wand
- Apply as normal

Massage Oil

Feminine Message Oil Blend

This recipe is profoundly relaxing and exudes a floral, feminine aroma.

How To:
- Add 4 drops Clary Sage
- 4 drops Geranium
- 2 drops Lavender
- 1 ounce Sweet Almond
- Mix into your favorite carrier oil

Masculine Message Oil Blend

How To:
- 4 drops Frankincense
- 2 drops Lavender
- 4 drops Sandalwood Australian
- 1 ounce Sweet Almond
- Mix into your favorite carrier oil

Nail Care

Nail scrub

It is very common to get a mild infection after pushing back, and snipping off your extra cuticles. Instead try this fabulous way to remove unwanted cuticles gently.

How To:

- Create a smooth paste of: three parts baking soda to one part water
- 2 drops Tea Tree EO
- Dip a nail brush into the paste
- Gently rub in a circular motion over your hands and fingers
- Rinse with warm water
- Then apply nail polish as usual

Cuticle Oil

Get rid of hangnails and dry, cracked cuticles with this cuticle oil.

How To:

- Fill a 15ml bottle with Olive Oil
- add 10 drops of Frankincense EO
- Apply to cuticles and massage in

Strengthen Nails

How To:
- Add 1 drop of melaleuca (tea tree) EO
- 1/4 teaspoon of olive oil
- Apply directly onto your nails
- Massage in to strengthen them

Outdoors

Ice Cooler Odor Eliminator

Avoid that musty, moldy smell that camping equipment forms after storing.

How To:
- Add 10 drops of any citrus EO to a box of baking soda
- Shake well
- Sprinkle a bit of baking soda into your clean and dry cooler, thermos, and even tents before storing them away

Patio Furniture

How To:
- Mix 1 small box baking soda with 20 drops of your favorite EO
- Scatter baking soda under chair cushions
- Store for the winter or shake off and use for the summer

Patio Furniture Sparkling Clean

How To:
- Mix 1 small box of baking soda
- 1 Tbsp. of natural dishwashing soap
- 20 drops of pine, lemon, lemongrass or eucalyptus EO
- 1 gallon of warm water

- Dip sponge or cloth into mixture and apply
- Rinse well

Grill Cleaning

Keep your grill clean all summer long.

How To:
- Mix ½ cup baking soda
- 10 drops Oregano EO
- Start scrubbing the grate
- Then rinse well

Parasite Removal

Parasite Detox Drink

How To:
- Take this solution before bed, without food or drinks other than water
- Dissolve a quarter teaspoon of soda in a glass full of warm water
- Add 1 drop of Peppermint EO
- Drink
- Repeat every night for three days

Pesticides Non-Toxic

Pantry Bug Repel

How To:
- Wipe down shelves with a mix of white vinegar and 2 drops of EO
- Try Citronella, Eucalyptus, Tea Tree or Peppermint EO

Ant & Spider Spray

Ingredients:
- 1 small spray bottle
- Distilled water
- 2 tablespoons of witch hazel
- 12 drops of Peppermint EO

How To:
- Take your small spray bottle and fill it 3/4 full of distilled water
- Add 2 tablespoons of witch hazel to the spray bottle
- Then add 12 drops of Peppermint EO
- Shake it well and spray away

Repel Ants

How To:
- Open a box of baking soda
- Place 5 drops of Peppermint EO on to lid
- Keep under sinks and cabinets to repel ants

Mosquito Bracelet

Make your own bug bracelet.

How To:
- Braid cotton fabric or leather
- Wrap around your wrist
- Put a few drops of Citronella, Lemongrass, or Lavender EO directly onto the outside of bracelet
- Wear bracelet to repel mosquitos

Pets

Waterless Dog Bath

Dry clean your dog! It works the same as dry shampoo for humans. The Lavender also provides extra flea protection.

How To:
- Mix 1/4 cup baking soda with 2 drops Lavender EO
- Just sprinkle your pooch with baking soda
- Massage it in
- Brush it out
- It's completely non-toxic and safe for your furry friend

Kitty Litter Solutions

How To:
- Mix 3 drops Lemongrass EO and 1 cup baking soda
- Shake well
- Sprinkle baking soda in the empty kitty litter box
- Add litter on top

Pet Tooth Paste

How To:
- Mix together ½ cup of baking soda
- ½ cup of coconut oil
- 8-10 drops Peppermint EO

- Put the paste on the toothbrush
- Brush gently

FYI: Your pet cannot spit out the extra, so be sure to use a little at a time.

No Bug Zone

How To:
- Mix together baking soda and a few drops of Lavender EO (you can also use Peppermint EO)
- Surround your pet's food and water bowl to keep pests away.

Deodorize Pet Bedding

Eliminate odors from your pets bedding.

How To:
- Mix together baking soda and 5-10 drops of Lavender EO
- Sprinkle on all pet bedding
- Leave for 2-24 hours
- Vacuum or shake out well

Home-Made Flea Collar

A flea collar is a great way to ward off fleas and is free of all toxins

Ingredients:
- Add 3-5 drops of Cedar or Lavender EO

- 2 tablespoons of water
- ½ tsp. of Olive Oil
- Bandana OR your dog's collar
- Eyedropper (optional)

How To:
- Add together
- Apply 8 drops of the mixture to a bandana or collar
- Rub the sides of the fabric together
- Reapply oil mixture to the collar once a week

Flea Spray

This flea spray is an easy way to prevent fleas as well as ticks from hitching a ride on your dog. It also makes their hair shimmer.

Ingredients:
- 1 cup apple cider vinegar
- 1 quart fresh water
- 2-3 drops of Lavender or cedar EO
- 1 medium/large sized spray bottle

How To:
- Add all ingredients together
- Mix with 1 quart of fresh water
- Fill your spray bottle, and mist your dog
- Do not spray directly at their face
- To get around the neck and behind the ears, dampen a soft cloth with the mixture and wipe it on
- Lightly spray their bedding and resting areas

Flea Bath

Wash your pooch to kill fleas on the spot.

Ingredients:
- 1/2 cup of freshly squeezed lemon juice
- 1 ½ cups of fresh water
- 1/4 cup of shampoo (plant based - natural)
- 2 drops of Lemongrass EO
- 2 drops of Cedarwood EO

How To:
- Stir together
- Bottle the remainder and use every few days until fleas are gone
- Make sure that you message the mixture deep into the hair and rinse well

Reed Diffuser

Make Your Own Reed Diffuser

Follow these 10 steps to make your own reed diffuser. Then choose an Essential Oil Combination below.

1. Add 1/4 cup of a light oil like apricot kernel oil or safflower oil to a glass measuring cup
2. Add 2 Tbsp. of alcohol to the measuring cup. Cheap vodka works great!
3. Add 15 drops essential oil
4. Stir well
5. Pour the oil and alcohol mixture into the vase
6. Bundle the reeds and insert them into the neck of the vase
7. It will take a few days for the reeds to absorb the oil
8. Flip sticks every few days to refresh scent
9. replace the oil-alcohol mixture once it evaporates and replace the reed sticks about once a month

Essential Oil Combination – Reed Diffuser

- 8 drops Eucalyptus + 8 drops Spearmint
- 5 drops Grapefruit + 5 drops Orange + 3 drops Lemon + 1 drops Bergamot
- 3 drops Geranium + 8 drops Lavender + 5 drops Orange
- 10 drops Lavender + 7 drops Clary Sage + 7 drops Orange
- 5 drops Lemongrass + 5 drops Lavender + 6 drops Eucalyptus

- 7 drops Tangerine + 7 drops Spearmint + 7 drops Lemongrass
- 2 drops Geranium + 5 drops Lavender + 8 drops Lime
- 13 drops Lemon + 4 drops Frankincense + 4 drops Ylang Ylang
- 5 drops Lavender + 5 drops Lemon + 6 drops Rosemary
- 7 drops Lavender + 7 drops Lemon + 7 drops Peppermint
- 5 drops Lemon + 5 drops Lavender + 6 drops Grapefruit

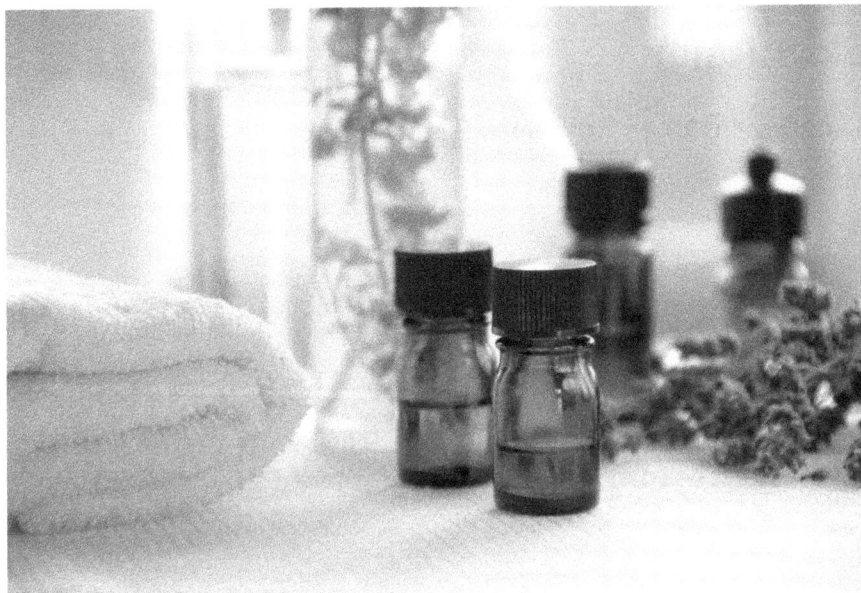

Skin Care

Facial Acne Relief

How To:
- Combine enough baking soda, water, and 1 drop of Tea Tree EO to make a creamy paste
- Apply the paste on the acne affected areas
- Let paste sit on your face for 2-10 minutes
- Rinse paste off thoroughly with warm water
- Repeat the process 1x per week

FYI: Baking soda may dry out the skin. Use a good moisturizer to keep skin hydrated.

Skin Toner

2-ingredient toner that removes makeup residue and tighten your pores.

How To:
- Add 2 drops of Tea Tree EO
- 1 ounce witch hazel
- Shake it up
- Then saturate a cotton pad and gently wipe your face using an upward motion from jawline to forehead (avoiding your eyes)

Damage Repair

This is an amazing Frankincense day and night cream for your face and neck.

Ingredients:
- 1 cup cocoa butter
- 1/4 cup coconut oil
- 2 Tbsp. jojoba oil
- 2 Tbsp. sweet almond oil
- 30-40 drops Frankincense EO

How To:
- Bring cocoa butter to room temperature or slightly soft
- Combine softened cocoa butter, coconut oil, jojoba oil, and almond oil in a mixing bowl
- Place the bowl into your fridge until it starts to harden
- Then whip the oils with a mixer
- Slowly add Frankincense until mixed well

- Use small amount on your neck and face day and night
- Keep in a cool place in a glass container

Night-Time Face Care

Ingredients:
- 1 teaspoon of Evening Primrose oil
- 2 drops of Geranium oil
- 1 drop Lavender oil
- 1 capsule of Vitamin E, with contents drained into mixture

How To:
- Mix the above recipe in a clean, amber bottle to keep protected from sunlight
- In the evening after cleansing, apply the blend to your face, paying particular attention to any areas of redness and wrinkles
- Let it soak in for at least 10 minutes before heading to bed

Skin Irritation Blend

For skin irritations.

How To:
- Add 1 tablespoon Sweet Almond oil
- 1 teaspoon Avocado oil
- 1 teaspoon of Evening Primrose EO
- 15 drops Helichrysum EO
- 5 drops Lavender EO
- 1 capsule of Vitamin E

- Mix well and apply as needed

Razor burn cream

How To:
- Add 3 oz. coconut oil
- 1 tsp grapeseed Oil
- 8 drops Peppermint EO
- 3 drops Lavender EO
- 3 drops Tea Tree EO
- Mix with an electric mixture until you get a white fluffy texture
- Apply all over your skin after shaving

Soothing Sunburn Cream

How To:
- Add 4 tsp Aloe Vera gel
- 15-20 drops Lavender EO
- Mix well
- Gently apply to sunburned skin

Chicken Pox – Hives – Measles

If you are suffering from chicken pox, hives, or measles then try this bath soak. It will reduce the severe itchiness and stimulates healing.

How To:
- Run a warm bath

- Put in ½ cup of baking soda
- 5 drops Chamomile EO
- 5 drops Jasmine EO
- Soak in the tub until water cools
- Towel off when done

Splinter Remover

If you have a splinter that is too deep to be removed easily, this solution will force it out of your skin.

How To:
- Add a tablespoon of baking soda to a small glass of water
- 1-2 drops Tea Tree EO
- Soak the affected area 2x per day
- The splinter will be forced out within a few days

Hand Cleanser

This natural hand cleanser will scrub away dirt and neutralize odors.

How To:

- Add 1-2 Tbsp. of castile soap
- 15-25 drops of essential oil of your choice
- Add water to near top of dispenser
- Add pump lid
- Shake

Popular EO for Hand Soap:

Blood Orange – Blood orange reduces inflammation, is anti-septic and works to gently detox through the skin. It leaves your hands feeling and smelling clean.

Lemon – Lemon oil is naturally anti-bacterial, safe, gentle cleanse, a fresh citrus scent, and it improves skin conditions.

Peppermint – Peppermint has a cooling effect on the skin, also known to reduce itchiness and repels bugs.

Sleeping Aid

Pillow Dreams

Experience a restful night with this EO remedy.

Ingredients:
- 5 drops Bergamot EO
- 10 drops Chamomile Roman EO
- 5 drops Clary Sage EO

How To:
- Mix this blend
- Store in a glass bottle
- Put a few drops on your pillow each night for a restful sleep

Sore Muscles & Inflammatory Bath Soaks

These bath soaks are the best remedy for reducing entire body inflammation, relieve aches and pains, muscle cramps, muscle relaxer, remove toxins, a natural emollient for your skin, and reduces lactic acid build-up. Feel the magic of body and mind!

Sore Muscles

Ingredients:
- 3 cups Epsom salts
- 1 Tbsp. sweet almond oil
- 3 drops Lemongrass EO
- 3 drops Basil EO
- 3 drops Lavender EO
- 2 drops Lime EO
- 6 drops Wintergreen EO
- 6 drops Rosemary EO
- 6 drops Peppermint EO
- 4 drops Bergamot EO
- 4 drops Douglas Fir EO
- 4 drops Ginger EO
- 2 drops Marjoram EO
- 5 drops Lavender EO
- 4 drops Rosemary EO

How To:
- Put the Epsom salts into a quart sized mason jar
- Drip the essential oils onto the salts and add the carrier oil
- Close tightly and shake well
- Use 1/4 to ½ of the jar in hot bath water

- Soak for at least 20 minutes to relieve soreness from overworked muscles

Eucalyptus Soak

Soak in this Eucalyptus bath for purifying, oxygenating, energizing and detoxifying effects. Works wonders for general sore muscles, feet, upper and lower back pain.

Ingredients:
- 1 Cup Epsom Salts
- 1/4 Cup Sea Salts
- 1/4 Cup Baking Soda
- 3 drops each of Eucalyptus EO
- 3 drops Rosemary EO

How To:
- Mix all ingredients together in a small bowl
- Begin filling bathtub with hot water
- Place the mixture under the faucet as it is filling
- Soak for at least 20 minutes
- Do a quick rinse
- Pat dry with a towel
- Go bed immediately as you may become very drowsy

Sport Soak

Refreshing salt soak for sore muscles caused by a heavy workout.

Ingredients:

- 5 drops Lavender EO
- 2 drops Peppermint EO
- 2 drops Citrus EO
- 1 drops Clove EO
- 1 Tbsp. Jojoba EO

How To:

- Fill your bathtub
- Drop all EOs in water
- Soak for at least 20 minutes
- Do a quick rinse
- Pat dry with a towel
- Go bed immediately as you may become very drowsy

Stinky Stuff Neutralizer

Magic Smell-Good Bars

How To:
- Mix 2 cups of baking soda
- 1/4 cups distilled water in mixing bowl
- Now add 4 drops Lavender EO or any EO of your choice in another 1/4 cup of distilled water
- Combine all ingredients
- Pour into a silicone mold or muffin pan
- Let sit for 24-48 hours, until dry and solid
- Place anywhere you want to neutralize smells

FYI: Great for behind toilets, trash area, inside laundry hamper, by the cat box, in closets, drawers, or shoe area.

Toothpaste & Mouth Care

Why Use Natural Toothpaste?

Store-bought Toothpaste Ingredients:
- Fluoride: Fluoride interferes with thyroid hormones. fluoride does come with a warning to call the poison control center immediately if ingested.
- Triclosan: A chemical used in antibacterial soaps and products. Triclosan was found to affect proper heart function.
- Glycerin: Glycerin is a sweet, colorless liquid and some research says it can coat teeth and prevent them from benefitting from minerals in saliva.
- Surfactants: Many toothpastes contain surfactants like sodium lauryl sulfate, which gives toothpaste its foam and lather. It can cause mouth ulcers and canker sores.
- Artificial: Colors/dyes or synthetic flavors.

Natural Toothpaste

Ingredients:
- 1/2 cup coconut oil
- 2-3 Tablespoons of baking soda
- 2 small packets of stevia powder
- 15 drops of peppermint or Cinnamon EO
- 5 drops Myrrh EO

Instructions:
- Slightly soften coconut oil
- Mix in other ingredients and stir well
- Put mixture into small glass jars
- Let cool completely

Whitening Toothpaste

If you need to use whitening toothpaste, use this non-toxic recipe. It will whiten your teeth without experiencing the painful sensitivity that comes with store-bought tubes.

Ingredients:
- 1/4 cup Calcium Carbonate Powder
- 3 Tablespoons Xylitol powder
- 1/4 cup MCT oil (plus more for thinning if needed)
- 10-20 drops Spearmint EO (add more as needed)

How To:
- Make sure the xylitol is finely ground and not coarse
- Mix all ingredients by hand or with a blender until incorporated
- Store in a glass jar and use as you would regular toothpaste

FYI: Xylitol is naturally coarse, use the blender to make the powder fine. In case you do not know what MCT oil is, it is derived from coconut oil or palm oil. The process is unique and provides a great base for this toothpaste.

Mouthwash

This natural mouthwash kills germs, freshens breath and heals sores.

How To:
- Mix ⅛ cup witch hazel
- ½ cup Aloe Vera juice
- 1 cup distilled water

- 10 drops of Peppermint EO
- Add all to a jar and shake well

Clean Your Toothbrush

Many people overlook the need to clean their toothbrushes. However, many disgusting things thrive on this tiny wet bristle.

How To:
- Add 1/4 cup baking soda
- 10 drops Peppermint or Lemon EO
- 1/4 cup water
- Mix well
- Let toothbrushes stand overnight
- Rinse and use the next morning

Mouth Appliance Cleaner

Soak oral appliances, like retainers, mouthpieces and dentures, in this amazing solution.

How To:
- Dissolve 2 teaspoons of baking soda
- With 2 drops Lemongrass EO
- Into a glass or small bowl of warm water

Canker Soar Solution

This really goes to work treating painful canker sores on the lips, gums, tongue and throat.

How To:
- Mix 1 tablespoon of water
- 1 drop Clove EO
- 1 teaspoon of baking soda
- Make a fine paste
- Apply to affected areas in the mouth
- Let sit until dry
- Gargle with warm water until mouth is rinsed
- Repeat the same process once daily

Upset Stomach

Baking Soda + Warm Water + Lemon

This process helps to soothe the stomach and chest.

How To:
- Add 1 teaspoon of baking soda to 1 cup of warm of water
- 1 drop Lemon EO
- Mix together and drink
- Provides relief within 10–15 minutes
- Repeat every 3 hours, if upset stomach persists

Baking Soda + Lemon + Peppermint Leaves

The peppermint leaves are uplifting and the lemon adds a touch of sunshine.

How To:
- Add ½–1 teaspoon of baking soda
- 1 teaspoon of lemon juice
- 1-2 drop Peppermint EO
- ½ cup of water
- mix it well
- Add small ice cubes

Urinary Tract Infection

Ease Urinary Pain

How To:

- Mix 1 tbsp. baking soda
- 3-5 drops Lemon EO in 32 ounces of water
- Drink the mixture to reduce the pain of a urinary tract infection

Vehicle & Mechanical

Dead Bugs

It may be one of the most best cleaning solution to remove insect carnage from unpainted car surfaces like bumpers and windshields. Also use on headlights and yellowing plastic.

How To:
- Create a creamy paste by mixing baking soda and water together
- Add 2 drops Wild Orange or Lavender EO
- Make as much or as little of this paste as you would like
- Add a little dish soap
- Gently scrub the areas of concern with a sponge, microfiber or washcloth
- Rinse well

Diffuse as You Drive

You can make a simple car diffuser from just a clothespin, hot glue and felted balls.

How To:
- Glue felt balls onto a wooden clothespin
- Whenever your car smells musty drip a drop or two of essential oils onto the balls and then clip it over your air vent

Car Wash

A perfect solution for cleaning entire car, tires, windows, floor mats and vinyl seats.

How To:
- Add ½ cup of baking soda in a half gallon of warm water
- Add a squirt of dish soap
- 10-20 drops of Lemon, Lemongrass or Orange EO
- Gently scrub the entire car
- Rinse well
- Dry with cloth or microfiber towel

Tires & Hubcaps

How To:
- Mix one-half cup baking soda
- 1 tablespoon of dish soap
- 10 drops Lemon EO
- 2 cups of warm water into a small bowl
- Use a soft sponge or towel to gently scrub the tires and hubcaps
- Rinse well

Deodorizing Cars

How To:
- Mix 5 drops of your favorite Essential Oil to 1 cup baking soda
- Sprinkle directly on the fabric and carpets

- Let sit for 1-24 hours
- Vacuum well

Wasted EO Bottles

Reuse Ever Last Drop

Inside the empty EO bottle is a small amount of oil. Turn the remainder into a fantastic bath salt.

How To:

- Tip your empty bottle of EO down into a container of Epsom Salt
- The EO bottle will slowly drain into the salt
- Use the salt in your bath water

www.ingramcontent.com/pod-product-compliance
Lightning Source LLC
Chambersburg PA
CBHW022117280326
41933CB00007B/429